I0408419

Intermittent Fasting

*Unleash Your Body's Potential to Burn Fat and
Build Lean Muscle Fast, While Eating the
Foods You Love*

Kelvin Sprinkle

TABLE OF CONTENTS

Introduction

♥ Copyright 2017 by Kelvin Sprinkle- All rights reserved.

The follow eBook is reproduced below with the goal of providing information that is as accurate and reliable as possible. Regardless, purchasing this eBook can be seen as consent to the fact that both the publisher and the author of this book are in no way experts on the topics discussed within and that any recommendations or suggestions that are made herein are for entertainment purposes only. Professionals should be consulted as needed prior to undertaking any of the action endorsed herein.

This declaration is deemed fair and valid by both the American Bar Association and the Committee of Publishers Association and is legally binding throughout the United States.

Furthermore, the transmission, duplication or reproduction of any of the following work including specific information will be considered an illegal act irrespective of if it is done electronically or in print. This extends to creating a secondary or tertiary copy of the work or a recorded copy and is only allowed with express written consent from the Publisher. All additional right reserved.

The information in the following pages is broadly considered to be a truthful and accurate account of facts and as such any inattention, use or misuse of the information in question by the reader will render any resulting actions solely under their purview. There are no scenarios in which the publisher or the original author of this work can be in any fashion deemed liable for any hardship or damages that may befall them after undertaking information described herein.

Additionally, the information in the following pages is intended only for informational purposes and should thus be thought of as universal. As befitting its nature, it is presented without assurance regarding its prolonged validity or interim quality. Trademarks that are mentioned are done without written consent and can in no way be considered an endorsement from the trademark holder.

INTRODUCTION

Congratulations on downloading *Intermittent Fasting: Unleash Your Body's Potential to Burn Fat and Build Lean Muscle Fast, While Eating the Foods You Love* and thank you for doing so. By the end of your reading, it will be clear how beneficial the theory of fasting in this way will benefit your life in the long-term by making you both look and feel better than you ever thought possible.

The following chapters will discuss what specifics are essential to fast successfully and lose the unwanted pounds, without losing your sanity in the process. You will discover health benefits and also not need to prepare as many meals. After all, with such a busy lifestyle who can complain for less cleanup time in the kitchen? Your day will automatically be simplified without having all of the extra meals to prepare.

Think of the intermittent fasting plan as a schedule and not a diet. You need to consider it takes a time slot of about three to six weeks for your body to adapt to the plan. You can successfully drop the weight, but it is a continuous process.

Think of the plan as a method to place a new concept to hunger. Think of your intermittent fasting plan as an association of pride and success—not of hunger—desire—or even panic. You may be a little uncomfortable during the time your body adapts, but you will love the results.

There are plenty of books on this subject on the market, thanks again for choosing this one! Every effort was made to ensure it is full of as much useful information as possible; please enjoy!

CHAPTER 1

INTERMITTENT FASTING EXPLAINED

Using a plan of to improve your health, lose, weight, and simplifying your lifestyle is what intermittent fasting is focused upon in this informative book. As a beginner, you will discover it is important to adjust your eating patterns or habits.

What is Intermittent Fasting (IF)?

Several plans are used when you choose to encompass the program which includes two times each week, for twenty-four hours, or for sixteen hour fasting times. The process causes your levels of insulin to rise and fall as part of your essential cellular repair practices.

Fasting has been a part of some religious beliefs including Buddhism, Islam, and Christianity. Decades before this generation, the process may have been because of the unavailability of food resources. Moving forward to today's society, you have a choice to choose a suitable eating plan by eating and fasting periods that are split by the week or day.

You will be consuming fewer calories and losing belly fat as well as the weight. After you begin the new intermittent fasting process, you will discover it is much easier than most of the traditional methods for losing weight. It makes the long-term much simpler to reach the goals when you have a plan.

Have a Checkup Before You Begin Fasting Plans

Before you begin an intermittent fasting plan, you should check with your physician to be sure you are physically fit. These are some of the elements to consider:

- [ ] History of eating disorders
- [ ] Have diabetes
- [ ] If you are too thin/underweight
- [ ] Have low blood pressure
- [ ] Currently taking prescribed or non-prescribed medications
- [ ] Have issues with regulation of your blood sugar
- [ ] Female with amenorrhea history
- [ ] Female actively attempting to become pregnant
- [ ] Breastfeeding or pregnant
- [ ] History of eating disorders

Important Note: Keep in mind, nothing is considered risky or dangerous in intermittent fasting, but it is always best to be sure you are healthy before you make any major changes in your diet needs.

Remember the most common consequence using this procedure is hunger—not starvation. You might experience some mood swings and want to over-eat when you are on your days off, but the plans are healthy. You also, will not starve!

How Much to Lose on the Intermittent Fasting Plan

To reach your goals, you first need to understand how much weight you need to lose. You can use the chart below to calculate your goal weight:

Lifestyle Description	Individual Body Weight Multiplier (calories to pound ratio)
Extremely Active	18 to 19
Very Active	14 to 15
Moderately Active	12 to 13
Lightly Active	11 to 12
Sedentary	10 to 11

Once you have your diet plan in motion, you can begin to reach your desired goals.

Trick Your Body's Thinking Patterns

Intermittent fasting takes a lot of courage and determination. Begin by placing healthier foods in an area where you frequent. If special ingredients are listed in your plan, make each of them readily available, so you won't be tempted to grab the gallon of ice cream from the freezer when you are in a rush. These are a few of the tips to help keep your plan in motion:

☐ **The Plate:** Use a smaller plate to make it appear to be more food than is acceptable. Research has proven if you switch from a 12" plate to a 10" plate—over one year—you will reduce your consumption by approximately 22%. This is a much simpler way to get the smaller servings without feeling deprived. It works!

☐ **The Glass:** Consuming less of the beverages you don't want on your fasting plan can be accomplished if you consider using a tall glass. Try it the next time you want to have a tumbler of soda instead of using the fat/short one. They may contain the same amount of liquid, but it is a trick of your mind that works.

☐ **Make the Plate Pretty**: Try using contrasting colors instead of a color that blends. For example, when you have some dark green veggies—try using a light colored plate. It has been studied with several experiments that your brain has difficulty distinguishing the size of the portions unless there is a contrasting background. It is a simple feat. Try it; you might be surprised!

☐ **The Package:** If your family chooses not to join you with your new intermittent fasting routine, try wrapping the foods differently. You have heard the adage of out of sight and out of mind. It is the same when you are fasting. Wrap the foods you are not allowed to have in an opaque container or foil. Use plastic wrap on the foods you are allowed on your plan.

Simple Guidelines to Follow

☐ **Stay in Control:** Depending on which method you choose for your intermittent fasting routine, you need to ask the question if you can follow the crucial diet plans involved to keep your food intake at proper levels. If you are attempting to achieve a 500 calorie debit daily, you have to keep your appetite under control, because a single missed meal won't provide a generous window for the next meal.

☐ **Keep a Calorie Tally Record:** You must keep an accurate record of your calorie intake because if you are not careful, you can easily overeat at mealtime. If your goal is to work off more calories than you consume to lose the 1 pound of weight you want to lose each week.

☐ **Stay with the Chosen Plan:** you need to get into the habit of setting a regular schedule for your fasting plan. Once your body adjusts to the specific method, it will become confused if you try another plan. For example, if you are on the 5:2 plan and switch to the 16:8 plan, your body will stop the weight loss until it can readjust to the new plan. You will lose valuable time by switching. Consistency is essential for a successful fasting plan.

Overview: The Basics of Adult Nutrition and Calorie Needs

You need to understand what your daily calorie needs will be to adopt a realistic diet plan and maintain a new desirable weight. The use of an adult BMI and Calorie Calculator will be an essential tool if the calories are not indicated in the recipe. Most products you purchase will have ingredient panels listing the counts, so you will have a general idea of how to plan your menu around your intermittent fasting plan.

You will need to enter your sex, height, weight, and age into the calculator. You will also need to provide the calculator with your daily activity schedule (such as daily—more than an hour—less than an hour—or rarely. The BMI will indicate your BMI score and the amount of calories necessary to maintain your current body weight. It will make your goals simpler to map by providing you with the tallies from your calculations to lower your counts.

Maintain a Healthy Diet Plan

The components for a healthier eating pattern using intermittent fasting methods will account for all of the beverages and foods within a suitable calorie level. A good plan for a healthy fasting pattern will include the following:

- ☐ Whole Fruits
- ☐ Oils
- ☐ Grains (a minimum of half should be whole grains)
- ☐ Protein foods such as eggs, poultry, lean meats, seafood, nuts, seeds, and soy products.
- ☐ Varied veggies from all of the main subgroups include— starchy legumes (peas and beans), red and orange, dark green and others.

Health concerns in the United States are focused on fundamental elements that should be limited when using the intermittent fasting diet plan. They recommend you do the following:

- ☐ Consume less than 10% of your daily calories from saturated fats.
- ☐ Eat less than 10% of your daily intake of calories from added sugars.
- ☐ Sodium consumption should be less than 2,300 mg (milligrams).
- ☐ Moderation must be accompanied if you consume alcohol products. You should have no more than one daily if you are a woman and only two each day if you are a man.

How Fasting Changes the Body

Your cells can modify your genes and begin significant repair process such as these:

- ☐ **Cellular Repair:** Your cells start to remove and digest the older/debilitated proteins that develop inside of your cells with a process called autophagy.

- **Gene Expression:** The functions of genes are altered regarding protection and continued existence alongside disease.

- **Insulin:** Lower insulin levels are improved as the diet produces sensitivity and levels stored in your body that make body fat more manageable.

- **HGH or The Human Growth Hormone:** Two samples of how the growth hormones will climb sharply with increased levels of five times the regular speed are from fat loss and muscle gain are two

The changes which occur are foremost weight loss tools because each step leads to a spontaneous decline in your intake of calories. The discharge of noradrenaline increases as a fat burning hormone.

Scientifically Proven

Your metabolic rate is increased with short-term fasting because of the hormonal changes ranging in categories of 3.6% to 14%. Studies have established weight loss after three to twenty-four weeks on the intermittent fasting program to maintain losses of 3.0 to 8.0%. In comparison to other studies on weight loss, these are high percentages that cannot be ignored.

In the same studies, many of the individuals lost 4.0 to 7.0% of his/her waist circumference. This is an indication of how the harmful buildup of belly fat can cause disease and other issues around your organs. You have to consider these results are from eating fewer overall calories, and not binging during the days off. You have to maintain a sensible eating program.

Benefits of Intermittent Fasting

Losing weight and building muscle are two of the main benefits created by intermittent fasting. You may have difficulty finding enough time in your busy routine to be concerned with preparing a healthy breakfast every day. Think of the money you can save in the long-term without all of the additional meals your consume. It might sound impossible to skip a meal or go for a day without eating a substantial meal, but it just takes forming a new pattern and adjusting your habits.

Health Benefits

Other than weight loss, you can receive benefits from intermittent fasting in many other ways. You will live a longer life from achieving an extended fasting state and diverting your energy while improving your biological functions.

Just remember, the plan will not in any way cause you to starve. The emergency signals transported by your body is simply that—a signal. The fasting state your body is experiencing will diminish once your body adjusts to the diet method of intermittent fasting you choose to take.

These are some of the crucial elements to consider:

- **Brain Health:** Your brain hormone—BDNF—also known as brain-derived "neurotropic" factor—is a protein that can aid in the growth of new nerve cells. It is also believed to provide protection against Alzheimer's and Parkinson's disease.

- **Cancer:** Studies using animals have suggested intermittent fasting can be beneficial in the prevention of cancer.

- **Heart Health:** The blood triglycerides, LDL cholesterol, insulin resistance, and blood sugar can be reduced using this plan. Each of these presents a huge risk element for heart ailments or disease.

- **Inflammation:** Chronic diseases are driven by inflammation and the fasting plans help to reduce the inflammation as proven by private studies. Your body will be capable of repairing, healing and recovering more quickly than without the diet plan.

- **Insulin Resistance:** Your blood sugar levels can be lowered by 3.0% to 3.6 as fasting insulin levels can also decrease as much as 20% to 31%. These figures indicate you should be better sheltered against type 2 diabetes as well as a more continuous level of mood and energy stages.

- **Anti-Aging:** The process has only been tested using animals, but the rats tested lived 36% to 83% longer than ones that were not fasting.

- **Lower Stress Levels:** The cortisol production is lowered.

- **Fatty Acid Oxidation:** Your body will burn more fat as energy with the oxidation process and will also provide quick weight loss.

Note: Each of these studies is in early stages. More research needs to be provided using human testing during the fasting process.

How to Boost Your Metabolism

With all of the hard work for your intermittent fasting, it is always good to know there are other ways to speed up the process at the same time. It is virtuous to know these are some of the specific foods you should eat to help the metabolism process of losing weight:

Protein-Rich Food Groups

Your body will need more energy to digest these products:

- ☐ Eggs
- ☐ Seeds and nuts
- ☐ Legumes
- ☐ Fish
- ☐ Meat
- ☐ Fish

The thermic effect of food is referred to as TEF which is the amount of calories required by your body to absorb/digest the nutrients received by your meals. The protein intake will also make you have a full feeling much longer, and possibly prevent you from overeating.

Essential Vitamins and Minerals

Zinc, iron, and selenium are essential for your healthy body functions. It is shown by research a diet low in these elements reduces the ability of the thyroid gland to produce crucial hormones. This process will significantly slow the metabolism down. It is best to eat seeds, nuts, legumes, meat and seafood.

Chili Peppers: The chemical found in chili peppers is called capsaicin which will boost your metabolism. The capsaicin will increase the fat and calories you burn during your intermittent fasting plan. Twenty research studies indicated you would lose/burn approximately fifty extra calories daily. However, now all researchers agree with the theory. At any rate, enjoy the chili peppers.

Pulses and Legumes: This food group includes peanuts, lentils, chickpeas, beans, and peas which are extremely high in protein levels in comparison to other plant foods. According to research studies, your higher protein counts will require your body to burn a larger amount of calories to digest them, versus the lower-protein foods.

Recent studies have indicated participants who consumed a legume-rich diet for eight weeks increased the metabolism rate and lost more than 1.5 times more weight versus the other controlled group of applicants.

Coffee: Your caffeine levels can help increase the metabolic rate by approximately 11%. Studies have shown consumption of a minimum of 270 mg of caffeine—about three cups of coffee—will burn away an additional 100 calories daily. The rates can surely boost your intermittent fasting as long as you leave it sugar-free.

Tea: Tea is offered as a good source of beverage because of the catechins in the tea conglomerate with the caffeine to help speed up your metabolism. The catechins are an antioxidant and a type of natural phenol which is from the chemical family of flavonoids. An additional 100 calories can be burned daily to increase your metabolism by four to ten percent with the use of green and oolong tea. The effects may be different with each fasting participant.

Irregular Fasting

If you have become interested in intermittent fasting but are not sure if you want to commit, you might begin by fasting in periods for 12-hour periods several times weekly; just to see how your body reacts to the changes. You won't see the same effective results as with one of the specially prepared methods, but it will give you an idea of what to expect if you begin the process in the future.

As time passes with the new plan, you will become more willing to try one of the specific plans described in this book. The next time you are in the right mindset, you can begin and get the plan to stick forever. You will lose the weight once you find a plan that works for you.

6 Popular Intermittent Fasting Plans

The best option is to research the plans until you discover which one will best suit your circumstances. As popularity of the fasting plans performed intermittently over the past several years; they have been categorized into six popular methods including:

- ☐ Method 5:2
- ☐ Method 4:3
- ☐ Eat-Stop-Eat
- ☐ Method 16:8
- ☐ Alternate-Day Fasting
- ☐ The Warrior Diet

These methods will be thoroughly explained in the following chapters.

CHAPTER 2

METHOD 5:2 AND 4:3

For this plan, you would eat a regular diet for five days. For the remaining two days, you will eat approximately 500 to 600 calories. The baseline of the calorie ingestion is 2,000 for women and 2,500 for men. A few famous names swear by the diet including Jennifer Aniston and David Cameron. These are some of the ways of how to manage the 5:2 diet plan; just remember carbs don't mix with your fasting days.

Experiment with Mealtime

☐ Test different eating times. It doesn't always have to be an early time of day when you aren't hungry. You can wait a bit longer if you wish.

☐ Change from eating three meals each day to two such as having brunch. It can combine the meals and save the calories. Try having brunch around 11 am and dinner at 7, or even a larger meal at 8 with your significant other.

Maximize the Flavoring and Minimize the Calories

☐ Soups are a respectable choice—also proven by research— because you remain full longer than just a modest serving of veggies on a plate.

- [ ] Flavor your foods with spices and herbs such as these—lemon juice or vinegar for salads or curry pastes or chili flakes in stews, baked beans, or soups.

- [ ] Go for the veggies and salads with smaller servings of fish, eggs, lean meat, or tofu.

Use Fresh Ingredients

- [ ] Not only are you eating better and healthier products, but also most fresh ingredients are less expensive. Search for seasonal produce for the most savings.

- [ ] Search for items such as a tomato that have ripened that would make a yummy treat with a bit of your special herbs and balsamic vinegar. You could also add it to some soup.

- [ ] During the winter months, experiment with butternut squash or parsnip—roasted—with low-fat feta—or in soup.

- [ ] Cut some peppers in half and stuff them with cream cheese, tuna, or similar ingredients and grill them. You can add an egg to the mix for a taste challenge.

Food for the Fasting Days

- [ ] Berries and natural yogurt
- [ ] Plentiful veggie portions
- [ ] Baked or boiled eggs
- [ ] Low-cal 'cup' soups
- [ ] Other soups: vegetable, tomato, miso, cauliflower
- [ ] Lean mean or grilled fish

☐ Tea or black coffee

☐ Water (sparkling or still)

The 4:3 Diet Plan

Health benefits include asthma relief, reduction in heart arrhythmias, insulin resistance, menopausal hot flashes, seasonal allergies, and much more. After twelve weeks of fasting using the 4:3 method; these are the results from a small study group:

☐ Fat mass reduction: 3.5 kg with no muscle mass changes

☐ Body weight reduction: Over 5 kg

☐ Increased LDL particle size

☐ Reduced blood levels: 20% reduction of triglycerides

☐ Leptin levels: 40% decreased

☐ Levels CRP: Reduced levels (inflammation marker in your body)

How the4:3 Diet Plan is Different from the 5:2 Plan

The 5:2 intermittent fasting choices are much simpler than the 4:3 plan because you are more restricted. You will be intermittently fasting for three out of the seven days. You should not eat processed/sugary/refined foods for four of the days. If you do, your body will crave the supplementary fatty acids you need to thrive.

If you consume junk on those four days, you will defeat the purpose of the plan. Just remember, not to over-indulge. As you train your body by eating a well-planned diet; your body will adjust to the routine, and you won't feel as hungry.

The 4:3 plan acclaims you skip the morning meal, and it recommends you check your weight daily. However, this can be disheartening if your weight fluctuates.

A sample plan for the 4:3 method of weight loss is as follows:

Breakfast: Eat nothing.

Lunch: Leek, lentil, or chicken soup with a snack such as a small tangerine

Dinner: A side salad using lemon juice as the dressing with some salt, pepper, or similar seasonings along with a small lean fillet of grilled chicken

Snacks: Veggies or fruit

You can have a light breakfast if you enjoy a morning meal, but you will need to eliminate the snack during the day. You can also skip lunch, and have a larger breakfast. This is more challenging to follow than the 5:2 intermittent fasting plan because you have three days you can only consume 500 calories versus two days on the 5:2 diet.

Suggestions for the Fasting Days Using the 4:3 Method

- ☐ Drink an abundance of water.
- ☐ Drink coffee and tea for an additional boost.
- ☐ Consume a 400 calorie meal with a snack of 100 total calories.
- ☐ Chew sugar-free gum to fight the hunger spurts.

If you have a busy lifestyle, you can cheat once in a while with a low-calorie pre-packaged meal. (This is not a regular outlet.)

The point in both plans is to eat as much as you want and not feel deprived on the days you can eat normally—just do it in moderation, not over-indulgence.

CHAPTER 3

EAT-STOP-EAT

Once or twice each week, you will fast for twenty-four hours. As an illustration, you would eat dinner one morning and not eat again until the following morning. Most professionals say if you make it to twenty hours; it is okay.

To further condition your body, for two days eat about 2,500 calories if you are a man and 2,000 if you are a woman. After several regular eating days, attempt another fasting, and repeat the agenda.

Non-Fasting and Fasting Day Nutrients

For the days on an active fast, try not consume many calories. You can drink sparkling or plain water, diet soda, coffee, or tea. When the fast is complete, eat what you like using restraint. Enjoy plenty of veggies, fruits, and take advantage of the spices for variety.

Protein should be apparent using twenty to thirty grams of high-quality protein. Consume a total of one-hundred grams every four to five hours. You can use protein powders if needed. If you are gaining extra pounds during in between your fasting schedule, consider cutting back by approximately 10% on the amount of food you consume on non-fasting days.

Some individuals cannot 'hack' the plan and state it makes him/her less adaptable to enjoying time with friends at social gatherings. Many have issues of crankiness and headaches which can lead to the plan's failure.

With that said, the plan's benefits are overwhelming because you can judge your progress, and you choose to eat. It takes learning some self-control, but you can get it.

Note: Never fast two consecutive days. Also, you should not take the challenge more than two fasting days in one week.

Fluid Intake

With a strict plan such as this one, you must remain hydrated. You can drink plenty of clear liquids but where are the nutrients. On your fasting days, stick to apple juice water, broth, cranberry juice, ice pops, plain gelatin, black coffee or tea. This is okay since you will be fasting for twenty to twenty-four hours.

You can also enjoy foods including ice cream, skim milk, juice with pulp, or strained creamy soup. Try a whey protein supplemental shake or some low-fat frozen yogurt. These choices will provide some essential nutrients, fiber, as well as the necessary calorie counts. Just be sure to use low-calorie juices, ice cream, and a few ice cubes for a smoothie treat.

It is advisable to confer with your physician before you begin this or any other dieting plan. While you are fasting, you might need to discontinue any dietary supplements or medications. According to research at Vanderbilt University, daily liquid diets will provide you between 400 to 800 calories.

Additional Tips

With this fasting method, it is essential not to fall into a habit of fasting and binging because it will create havoc within your body. It is more than your body can handle since the cycle will only work for individuals who can practice control and moderate consumption of food. It is recommended by the professionals to perform resistance-style weight training on the days you aren't fasting.

Try a minimal yoga session or light cardio exercise if you are completely 'out of it' on your fasting days. Any more vigorous exercising could make it difficult to achieve the time allotment of your fasting schedule. Remember, at first—it is common to feel angered, anxious, fatigued, or have headaches. This will pass once your body adjusts to the new dieting plan.

Try to keep in mind; every single day you can successfully stay on your desired plan; is one more day toward your successful 30-day goal

CHAPTER 4

METHOD 16:8 OR THE LEANGAINS DIET PLAN

Another term for this plan is the 'Leangains protocol which implicates for a time slot of 8 hours you can eat a restricted diet and fast for the remainder time of sixteen hours for men, and fourteen hours for women. Hugh Jackman was the emblem used to discover the facts and make the headlines.

The 16:8 method for intermittent fasting is the most preferred method for weight loss—besides you will be sleeping for approximately eight of those fasting hours. On the remainder eight to ten hours, the meals should be slightly larger while still relatively health conscious. The fasting period allows for zero calorie consumption.

If you are overweight and have a sedentary lifestyle; you should avoid most of the starchy carbohydrates. You have to cram all of your calories in that time allotment to ensure the successes of the plan. Many individuals on the plan can fit two filling meals into the eight to ten-hour time frame or three regular meals if desired. The most important element once again is consistency.

A study was performed by the 'Obesity Society' stating if you have your dinner afore 2:00 p.m., your hunger yearnings will be reduced for the remainder of the day. At the same time, your fat-burning reserves are boosted.

No matter what you have heard about this plan, you will not be as hungry once you have the plan and your menu scheduled. That is the secret to a slimmer body, get the counts right. Another advantage is that you can begin the plate at any time that suits your schedule.

You can use these sample menus as a basis for your plan:

Day 1

- ☐ **Morning:** Tea, water, or coffee is allowed with a small amount of milk or heavy cream

- ☐ **Lunch:** Chicken Breast/black bean sauce, green veggies, and fruit.

- ☐ **Dinner:** Salmon and baked veggies with one potato. (If this is too much for one meal; break it in half and eat it later.

Day 2

Repeat Day 1

Additional Tips

Sugar Substitutes: Xylitol can replace sugar. Replace the coffee with black or green tea (advisable if you like the tastes).

Stay Hydrated: Drink plenty of tea, water, or coffee during the morning hours. It also helps prevent the pangs of hunger you will feel. If possible, replace the coffee with black or green tea.

Sleep: You need to have a full eight hours of sleep. It is advisable to avoid your cell phone and laptop (blue light) for up to an hour before you are ready to retire for the evening.

The Consistent Path

The goal is to set your eating schedule to the same time daily to program our body. If you vary the timing during the fasting plan, you hormones will be all over the place, resulting in your body holding onto the weight instead of detaching from the extra pounds.

It is also important to keep your protein on an even kilter throughout your fasting schedule. For women, it should remain at 55 grams daily, and for men, it should be in the area of 60 grams daily. If you consume the correct levels of protein and exercise regularly while taking in a steady amount of carbs, you should have all of the energy needed on a daily basis.

However, if you are less inclined to exercise you should focus on healthy fats while you minimize the carbs. Aim for approximately 0.7 grams of healthy fats for each pound of body weight daily. As with the other plans, it is best to avoid processed foods and unhealthy fats while searching for healthier—natural alternatives when possible. If you are not an avid exerciser, you also need to adjust your meals for the days you exercise to ensure you don't overeat accidently.

CHAPTER 5

EVERY-OTHER-DAY DIET PLAN

The alternate days using this plan was established by an assistant professor, Dr. Krista Varady, from the University of Illinois. Women should consume between 500 to 600 calories, and men need to consume more than 400 to 500 calories daily. However, on the feast day, you can eat anything you want and as much as you want.

The plan takes some planning since the diet begins between the hours of 12 noon and 2 pm. These are some of the items to make your day more enjoyable:

The following meal will supply you with roughly 475 calories—depending on the type of soup used.

- ☐ ½ cup cooked chicken cooked without the skin and topped/Lemon juice/Fresh-ground pepper

- ☐ Bowl of tomato or low-sodium vegetable soup

- ☐ 1 ¼ cups of fruit salad

For Men Only: You can have a whole-wheat roll (medium 96-calorie) for a total of 566 calories.

Prepare the salad with pears strawberries, mandarin orange segments, and melon.

Enjoy Lean Beef

Choose a lean piece of beef cut similar to sirloin or tenderloin steak, and enjoy some low-cal side dishes. The basics of the plan are charted for a woman; for a man—add 80 additional calories with a one-cup serving of asparagus with a teaspoon of olive oil for the topping.

For the remainder of the meal, enjoy a three-ounce seared steak with some onions. Top it off with a bit of blue cheese. Serve it with one cup of chard sautéed in 1 teaspoon of olive oil along with a ½ cup of polenta (cornmeal). Use some lemon juice for seasoning.

Substitute with Seafood

You need to consume some omega-3 fatty acids to remain heart-healthy. For men, boost the counts to 553 by enjoying one cup of kale that has been sautéed with olive oil for an additional 102 calories. Flavor the kale with crushed red pepper, red wine vinegar, and garlic.

As a woman (451 calories), enjoy three ounces of sautéed shrimp with jalapenos, garlic, onions, and some tomatoes (fresh and diced) on a bed of ½ cup of brown rice. Place it all in a six-inch corn tortilla. Also have ¼ of an avocado (chopped) for dessert.

The Choice of No Meat

Women can choose a meatless meal with 473 calories using a whole-wheat pizza crust. As toppings use some black beans, diced tomatoes, barbecue sauce, fresh corn, and shredded mozzarella cheese. Have a bowl of butternut squash soup made using ¾ cup of fruit sorbet and veggie stock.

Men can veg-out with one cup of cauliflower salad for an extra 48 calories using reduced-fat mayonnaise. He could also add ½ cup fruit such as blueberries, ½ cup yogurt if desired. It is best to use the lower fat plain yogurt with the meal.

A Week's Worth of Planning

The logic behind this weekly regimen example involves eating 300 calories on the low-calorie days but can increase to 400 calories if you have an exercise plan in motion. On the brighter side; women can eat 1200 to 1800 calories on the usual days.

The Low-Calorie Count Days

Day One:

Breakfast

1 small slice of deli meat

1 six-ounce glass of tomato juice

½ cup strawberries

Morning Snack Time

¼ cup mixed berries

1 tablespoon whey protein

Blend the ingredients with 3 ice cubes and a cup of water

Lunch

1-ounce low-fat cheese

½ cup of pickles

1-six-ounce cup of tomato juice

Afternoon Snacktime

1 tablespoon salad dressing (calorie-free) on one celery stalk

Dinner Time

Make an omelet using three egg whites, mushrooms, green peppers, and onions.

For Dessert have ½ cup of strawberries

Evening Snack

Whey protein smoothie is your savior to enjoy with a cup of mixed veggies.

Normal Calorie Counted Days

Day 2:

Breakfast

1 small banana

20 Blueberries

1 English muffin (whole wheat) with 2 ¼ teaspoons of peanut butter

2/3 cup fat-free yogurt

Morning Snacktime

3 saltines

1 reduced-fat string cheese stick

Lunch

3 tablespoons of hummus with tomato and lettuce

1 Whole wheat wrap

Dessert: 1 cup low-fat yogurt and ½ cup of applesauce

Afternoon Snacktime

15 almonds

Dinner

3 ounces—chicken breast

1 cup of broccoli and 2/3 cup of couscous

Evening Snacks

1 tablespoon peanut butter on 2 large graham cracker squares

Low Calorie Day

Day 3:

Breakfast Meal

½ fruit serving
1-ounce of protein
1 six ounce glass of tomato juice

Mid-morning Snack

¼ of a serving of fruit
Smoothie: Combine three pieces of ice + one cup of water with one tablespoon whey protein.

Lunch Menu

1-ounce of protein
1 six-ounce glass of tomato juice

Mid-afternoon Snack

Enjoy something under 50 calories.

Dinner Meal

No more than 100 calories—include protein, veggies, and fruit as a focus point

Normal Calorie Count Day

Day 4:

Breakfast Meal

20 blueberries
¼ cup banana
Whole wheat English muffin with 1 tablespoon of peanut butter

Mid-morning Snack

2 tablespoons of light cheese
3 rye crackers

Lunch

6 whole wheat crackers
1 cup of vegetable beef soup
1 piece fresh fruit

Mid-Afternoon Snack

5-6 medium strawberries
1-ounce dark chocolate

Dinner Menu

Steak and Peppers

Grill or broil:
1—four-ounce flank steak flavored with pepper and salt

Sauté Pepper Mixture:
2 teaspoons red wine
1 teaspoon olive oil
¼ cup onion sliced
¾ cup sliced bell pepper
1 tablespoon hoisin sauce

Instructions

Over a medium heat setting, sauté each of the ingredients listed using the teaspoon of olive oil.
After the flank steak is cooked to your preference, add the sautéed pepper mixture.

Calories: 267 per serving

CHAPTER 6

THE WARRIOR DIET

It is believed that the name of the diet is a reflection of the ancient ancestors who were natural nocturnal eaters. As a step up from the Leangains diet and as a variation of the daily fast; the Warrior Diet is a plan promoting one healthy meal daily—usually dinner. The method is parallel with the human 24-hour rhythm and can encourage excellent general health while removing the harmful toxins from your body. You should try to eat at least several hours before going to sleep for the night.

The Daytime Feeding Schedule

For the plan to be effective, you need to consume less food during the daytime hours. Eat small servings of veggies, fruits, and a protein such as a yogurt, whey protein, or kefir. Sidestep consumption of meats, grains, refined foods (pasta, corn tortillas, etc.) which lack the nutrient and are usually processed foods. Also, avoid sugary beverages and treats.

Every few hours, eat a small serving of protein or fruit. Eat green veggies such as celery, leafy greens, cucumbers, and peppers which are not restricted to your intake amounts.

Nighttime Feeding Frenzy

You can eat as much food as you wish but keep the correct food combinations. Enlist as many different aromas, colors, and textures to create new taste sensations for your evening meal. Eliminate or avoid using white vinegar. When you feel full or have satisfied your hunger or if you become more thirsty than hungry; it is time to stop eating.

Follow the Rules

Start off with your salad, protein, and veggies and complete the meal with a few fats or carbs. Take a short twenty-minute break after the protein and vegetables which will be a signal to your brain to recharge your appetite. If you are still hungry, continue your meal.

Organic foods are the best choices which will include grass-fed, free range, and hormone free animal products. Your eggs, dairy, and meat, as well as your fish consumption, should be a 'wild' catch.

Processed sugars are considered toxic on this diet plan.

You should also exercise as a critical step in your fasting plan. After your workout, consume 20 to 30 g of net protein with no additional sugar.

Guidelines for Success

Remember to plan your menus ahead of time to be sure you have the right combination of foods. Vegetables and protein will combine with your entire menu planning needs. Starch, sugar, and fat cannot conglomerate effectively.

Examples of the Right Combinations

Eggs and beans

Seeds and nuts

Eggs and potatoes

Berries and Whey protein

Cocoa nibs and peanut butter

Potatoes and peas

Nuts and wine

Cheese and wine

Rice and beans

Examples of the Wrong Combinations

Pasta and wine

Pasta and nuts

Raisins and nuts (trail mix)

Sugar and cream

Jelly and peanut butter

Jam and bread

Granola (honey nut)

Sour cream and potato

Sample Plan: Daytime Options

Early Morning: Tea, coffee, or cacao (no sugar) whole milk
Mid-morning: Vegetable juice or one fruit (8 ounces of berries)

Lunchtime: Salad with tomatoes, peppers, mixed greens, mushroom, onions,   sprouts, and cucumber
Dressing for the salad: Use a small amount of olive oil OR whey protein
Afternoon: Fresh Fruit OR Vegetable juice

Sample Plan: Nighttime Meal

For your one large meal of the day try some of the following food groups:

Protein: Eggs (cooked or poached), wild catch fish, organic cheeses such as goat and cottage

Cooked Veggies: Grilled or steamed cauliflower, broccoli, zucchini, onion, spinach, okra, and mushroom

Raw Veggies: Broccoli sprouts, salad greens, as well as red, yellow, and orange vegetables

Carbs: Use puree from butternut squash, carrots, Brussels sprouts, turnips, pumpkin, or cauliflower (steamed rooted veggies)

Use modest amounts of aged cheese, olive paste, parmesan cheese, or goat feta to top off your protein and vegetables. During the detox meals, you can also reduce stress with green tea and berberine. The berberine is a supplement to help unlock your metabolism to help balance your blood sugar levels during the detox diet plan.

The warrior diet is one of the most popular plans because it allows a sensible amount of snacks to the daily routing which makes it more appealing to beginners on the fasting path. The amount of energy will naturally get your body in the habit of burning fat for fuel.

CHAPTER 7

RECIPES FOR INTERMITTENT DIETING RESTRICTED: BREAKFASTS AND SNACKS

While you are attempting to lose weight on the intermittent fasting plan, you should not feel the need to be hungry no matter which of the procedures you decide to use. Some of the recipes call for grams which need to be converted to ounces. Use this <u>handy chart</u> to calculate the amounts.

This chapter is dedicated to some of the meals you can use. Each menu plan has a calorie count within the recipe.

Breakfast

Porridge

89 Calories: 25 g Porridge oats
10 Calories: ½ teaspoon honey
0 Calories: Water and Cinnamon

Instructions

Instead of milk, use some water to reduce the calorie count. For some additional flavor add just a pinch of cinnamon. You can also improve the meal with a few nuts if you add the calories to your plan.

Toast and Beans

55 Calories: 1 slice whole meal bread (small loaf size)
42 Calories: 50 g Baked beans

For a quick and low-cal choice, tempt your taste buds with this unique idea.

Fruity Breakfast Meals

Watermelon

The natural sugars are more beneficial than a cereal bar.
96 Calories: 300 g serving

Honey and Bananas

 10 Calories: ½ teaspoon honey
89 Calories: 1 small banana

Apricots and Yogurt

68 Calories: Two chopped apricots and 25 g Greek yogurt (low-fat)

Apricots, Greek Fat-Free Yogurt, and Mixed Berries

24 Calories: 3 tablespoons Greek yogurt
17 Calories: 1 Apricot
19 Calories: 50 g Raspberries
16 Calories: 50 g Strawberries
20 Calories: 50 g Blackberries
Total Calories: 96
Blend the ingredients for a yummy treat.

Greek Yogurt, Sultanas, & Almonds

24 Calories: 3 tablespoons Greek Yogurt (fat-free)
42 Calories: 1 tablespoon sultanas
28 Calories: 4 almonds (whole)
Total Calorie Intake: 94

Blueberries, Kiwi, & Greek Yogurt

42 Calories: 1 kiwi (chopped)
29 Calories: Blueberries (50g)
24 Calories: 3 tablespoons yogurt

Total Intake: 95 Calories

Mix all of the ingredients for a tasty meal.

Raspberry and Cranberry Smoothie

14 ounces/175 g raspberries
7 ounces cranberry juice
 3 ounces natural yogurt
Mint sprigs

For a quick and easy breakfast try this one packing 100 calories per serving.

Serves 4 to 6 people

Eggs for Breakfast

Plain Eggs

100 Calories: 1 large boiled egg

Add a slice of wheat toast with two small poached eggs for an 188 calorie delight.

Scrambled with Mushrooms

78 Calories: 1 medium egg
13 Calories: fresh chopped mushrooms (100 g)

Total Count: 91 Calories

Scramble the ingredients and enjoy!

Spinach Omelet

16 Calories: 60 g fresh spinach
78 Calories: 1 medium egg

Total Calorie Count: 94

Instructions

1. Simply, beat/whisk the egg and place in a frying pay.
2. When the bottom is cooked; add spinach to the top and grill.
3. If you want, you can some add herbs, salt, or pepper for additional flavoring.

Ham Omelet

19 Calories: 1 slice of ham/wafer sliced
78 Calories: 1 Egg (medium)

Prepare the ingredients as above.

Starchy Options

Bread with Honey

55 Calories: 1 slice bread (whole meal from a small loaf)
40 Calories: 2 teaspoons honey

Total: 95

Perfect Pancakes

2 eggs
1 1/3 cups milk (300 ml) 100 g all-purpose flour

Sunflower Oil

Instructions

Blend the ingredients, cook, and sprinkle with a splash of lemon juice.
114 Calories: Per serving

Total Servings: 4

Pancake Variation

2 whole eggs
1 ripe banana

Instructions

1. Simply blend the two ingredients until the bananas are completely mashed.
2. Gently grease a pan with a sprinkle of oil and add the batter.
3. Cook 20 to 30 seconds—flip—and enjoy.
4.

Calorie counts:

1 medium banana/118 g/105 calories
2 large eggs/100 g/156 calories

Total of 261 is not bad for these yummy delights!

In Advance: Fiber-Packed Cereal

If you have a busy lifestyle and always rushed in the morning, consider making this tasty breakfast bowl. It will serve 18 meals at 124 calories each.

100 g All-bran
300 g jumbo oats
50 g golden linseed
25 g wheat germ
140 g ready-to-eat apricots (chunked)
100 g dark raisins

Instructions

1. Blend all of the ingredients.
2. Ahead of time break down each of the units and store in airtight containers.
3. To serve: Add milk and let it soak. Grate some unpeeled apple over it for a flavor delight.

Note: The cereal can be safely stored for two months in the airtight container.

Snacks

Snack time doesn't always have to be boring. You can trick your mind by using the small plate mentioned earlier. Add some of these healthier choices to your intermittent fasting meal plan for weight loss. You will also notice the 'not so healthy' choices are higher calorie content, but that is the advantage of planning your menu before you are hungry. Each of these yummy delights will keep you going until lunchtime.

130 Calories: One square dark chocolate and a small banana
55 Calories: 10 g of 85% Dark chocolate
75 Calories: 3 Stuffed celery sticks with low-fat cottage cheese
96 Calories: 16 olives (green or black)
90 Calories: 1 Cup Cherries
29 Calories: 100 g Honeydew melon
42 Calories: 2 Satsumas/tangerine (The Christmas Orange)
90 Calories: 3 thin slices Pineapple
61 Calories: 100 g Grapes/ OR 100 Calories: 30 grapes
42 Calories: Sun-Maid Mini Box of Raisins
90 Calories: 25 Pistachio nuts
74 Calories: 10 Salted peanuts

Each Item Counts as 100 Calories:

31 Asparagus Spears
9—5" Spears of Broccoli
16 ribs Celery
12 Raw Brussels Sprouts
28 Baby Carrots
82 Red Kidney Beans
60 Raw Green Beans
43 Boiled or Steamed Okra Pods
100 Radishes
20 Sun-Dried Tomatoes

22 Cloves Garlic
100 Raspberries
5 Dried Figs
6 Dried Apricots
8 Cashew Nuts
10 Pringles Chips
21 Pretzels Unsalted Minis
4 Sardines in Oil Drained
13 Large Boiled or Steamed Shrimp
15 pieces Dry-Roasted Cashew Halves
Tasty Beverages Too Good to Pass Up!

Starbucks Grande Skinny Iced Latte: 96 Calories

Avocado—Chocolate Milkshake: 169 Total Calories/2 servings

Simply blend and enjoy:
1 ½ Cups skim milk
2 tablespoons cocoa powder
2 tablespoons brown sugar
½ ripe avocado
1 teaspoon vanilla extract

CHAPTER 8

FASTING RECIPES FOR INTERMITTENT LUNCHES

Lunchtime can be unpredictable, so here are some recipes to keep you satisfied.

Carrot—Cashew Toast

1 bacon slice/center-cut (cooked—crumbled)
1 slice toasted whole-grain bread (approximately 1 ounce)
1 large carrot
1 ½ tablespoons of Cashew butter
½ teaspoon apple cider vinegar
1 tablespoon freshly chopped flat-leaf parsley
½ teaspoon extra-virgin olive oil
Dash of black pepper and kosher salt to flavor

Instructions

1. Use a veggie peeler to shave a carrot into 1/3 cup of ribbons.
2. Mix the oil, parsley, carrot ribbons, and vinegar in a dish—toss.
3. Rest the ingredients for five minutes.
4. Butter the toast and top it off with the yummy mixture.

Calorie Intake: 271

Parmesan Zucchini

1 tablespoon Parmesan cheese (shredded)

1 cup sliced zucchini
10 butter spray squirts

Instructions

Use some foil to cover a cookie sheet.
Put the slices onto the pan and lightly spray the tops.
Broil just a few minutes until the cheese begins to brown.

One serving: 51.6 calories.

Cucumber Tuna Cups

1—1.5 ounce can tuna (water-packed)
1 medium peeled cucumber
1 tablespoon light mayonnaise
2 diced carrots

Instructions

1. **Form the Cups**: Slice the cucumbers cross-ways into one to two inch thick rounds.
2. Scoop the seeds out to use for filling or to throw away (your choice).
3. Mix the carrots, tuna, and mayonnaise—fill the cups.
4. Use diced carrots for the topping or the seeds' filling.
5. Chill and serve.

Recipe Yield: 6 Servings

Total Calories: 21.9 each

Cucumber and Tomato Salad

2 Cups chopped tomatoes

3 cups peeled/chopped cucumbers
¾ cup chopped purple onion
3 tablespoons fresh chopped cilantro
¼ cup fresh finely chopped parsley

Simply mix and enjoy for 25 calories

Serves 6

Pesto Beet Salad

3 beets
3 tablespoons olive oil
4 cloves of garlic
¼ cup pine nuts
5-ounces feta cheese
4 basil leaves

Instructions

1. Rinse and peel the beets—place them in foil with the garlic. (Wrap tightly.)
2. Sprinkle 1 tablespoon of the oil to the mix and bake for one hour at 400°F.
3. Remove and cool the beets.
4. Mix the basil, pine nuts, garlic, and the remaining 2 tablespoons of oil.
5. Blend until smooth in a food processor.
6. Chop the cooled beets into ½-inch cubes and mix with the pesto and feta cheese in a dish.
7. Blend to coat the beets and cool for four hours in the refrigerator until the flavors intertwine.
8. Yields: 12 servings

This tasty treat is 100 calories.

Tangy Pasta Salad

18 halved cherry tomatoes

200 g Rotini/fusilli pasta

4 tablespoons lite Italian dressing

1 tablespoon classic yellow mustard

3 tablespoons chopped parsley

8 slices pastrami

6 sliced gherkins

Instructions

1. Boil the pasta in salted water for ten minutes. Drain.
2. Blend the Italian dressing and mustard.
3. Add the tomatoes, parsley, gherkins, and pastrami.
4. Mix all items together.

Total Calories: 210

Butternut—Kale—and Chicken Salad

1 ounce (approximately ¼ cup) shredded chicken breast

1/8 teaspoon kosher salt

1 ½ cups kale

2 tablespoons red bell peppers (strips)

½ cups butternut squash (peeled, diced, and roasted)

1 ½ teaspoons extra-virgin olive oil

½ teaspoon molasses

1 teaspoon apple cider vinegar

¼ teaspoon Dijon mustard

2 tablespoons chopped pecans

Instructions

1. Mix the molasses, oil, vinegar, and mustard in a small dish.

2. Place the kale on a plate.
3. Top off with the rest of the ingredients.

This 5-minute miracle is worth 284 calories.

Snap Pea Salad and Halibut

4 Cups/12 Ounces Snap peas
1 lime cut into wedges
2 tablespoons olive oil
1 Small Red onion (thin slices)
1 tablespoon fresh lime juice
1 teaspoon fresh grated ginger
4—six-ounce halibut fillet pieces
1 tablespoon sesame seeds (if desired)

Instructions

1. Combine the ginger, lime juice, oil (1 tablespoon), and salt and pepper for extra flavor if desired.
2. Add the onion, peas (remove the strings), and sesame seeds. Toss to coat evenly.
3. Heat the remainder of the oil in a skillet using the med-high setting and add the halibut.
4. Cook approximately three to five minutes on each side (until opaque throughout the fish).
5. Serve with a wedge of lime.

Servings: 4

Calories: 313

Tuna Wrap

90 Calories: ½ six-ounce can of tuna

30 Calories: ¼ Cup Greek yogurt (non-fat)
130 Calories: 1 wrap (whole-wheat)
5 Calories: ½ Cup chopped celery
5 Calories: Small handful baby spinach
30 Calories: 3 Slices Red peppers (roasted)

Instructions

Combine the all of the ingredients and top it off with a squeeze of lemon for less than one calorie.

Total Calorie Intake: 382

Spicy Falafels

1 small onion
1 egg
400 g (14.11 ounces) can chickpeas
1 crushed clove garlic
1 teaspoon each ground cumin and coriander (see the note)
1 teaspoon dried mixed herbs
2 tablespoons vegetable or sunflower oil

Substitutes: You can use a handful of parsley for the mixed herbs and use more cumin if you do not want the coriander.

Instructions

1. Preheat a pan using low setting.
2. Add half of the oil, garlic, and onion.
3. Cook five minutes until the veggies are soft.
4. Add the spices and chickpeas—mash.
5. Stir in the dried herbs or parsley.
6. Add the egg and make into 6 balls/patties.
7. Add the remaining oil to the frying pan.

8. Cook each side for approximately three minutes on medium heat.
9. Serve with a salad, couscous, or pita bread. The falafels can be served hot or cold.

Serves 6 with 105 calories for each serving

Caprese Chicken

1 ½ cups halved grape tomato
1 cup cubed chicken breasts
1 ½ ounces fresh cubed Mozzarella

Combine the items for a delicious lunchtime special boasting 399 calories

Tomato and Cheese Sandwich

This yummy meal will provide you with a protein source with the cottage cheese combination.

120 Calories: 1 English muffin
40 Calories: ¼ Cup Cottage cheese (low-fat)
10 Calories: 2 Slices Tomato
68 Calories: ¼ Avocado
5 Calories: 1 Leaf Lettuce

You can add one tablespoon of chopped chives and garlic powder for less than one calorie each.

Total Calorie Count: 398

Artichoke Spinach Grilled Cheese

2 Ounces Deli turkey breast

2 slices wheat bread (reduced-calorie)\
½ cup fresh spinach
¼ Cup canned—chopped artichoke hearts
1 tablespoon light cream cheese
3 tablespoons part-skim—shredded mozzarella cheese

Instructions

1. Soften the cream cheese 30 seconds in the microwave for a spreadable consistency.
2. Mix the cheese, artichoke hearts, spinach, and flavor with salt and pepper.
3. Place the turkey between the slices of bread along with the spread mixture.
4. Use a skillet to cook the sandwich until toasty brown.

This is a yummy and simple sandwich that packs in 285 calories, but it is delicious.

Slow Cooker—Pork Au Jus

6 Cups Water
5 Pound Boneless pork loin
2 Au Jus packets

Instructions

1. For a great lunchtime treat; place the pork into a slow cooker at night.
2. Let it simmer eight hours on the low setting.

Total Calories: One Serving = 4 Ounces

Veggie Burgers Hawaiian Style

100 Calories: 1 Veggie burger patty
90 Calories: 1 Whole-wheat bun
25 Calories: 1 Round of pineapple
15 Calories: 2 tablespoons BBQ sauce
68 Calories: ¼ Avocado (mashed)
5 Calories: Alfalfa sprouts (handful)
Total Calories: 380

Note: Mayonnaise is substituted with the avocado since it is full of mono-saturated fats which are a healthy part of your diet plan.

Mint—Carrot—& Orange Soup

700 g carrots (peeled/thinly sliced)
2 tablespoons fresh chopped mint
32-ounces light vegetable stock
1½-2 tablespoons butter
1 large crushed garlic clove
1 large onion
4-Ounces orange juice

Instructions

1. Place the butter, onions, carrots, and garlic in a medium pan.
2. Cover and place on low heat approximately 12 minutes.
3. Pour the stock into the mixture and simmer 20 to 30 minutes.
4. Set aside to cool.
5. Strain the vegetables and save the liquid.
6. Blend the veggies until smooth.
7. Add the retained liquid until the mixture easily rotates in the blender/processor.
8. Add the mint and juice and salt if preferred.

Note: If you desire a smooth texture, push the pureed veggies through a sieve.

You may use a food processor or a blender for this recipe.

Total Calories: 120

Total Servings: 4

Black Bean Tacos

¾ cup drained black beans (canned for simplicity)

1/3 cup salsa (from the jar)

1. Cook the ingredients about five minutes in a small pan.
2. Three six-inch corn tortillas will complement the meal at 352 calories.

3-Ingredient Turkey Taco

1 ¼ Pounds—lean ground turkey
2 teaspoons seasoning mix
¼ cup water
12 corn tortilla shells

Instructions

1. Use a non-stick cooking spray in a skillet—preset on med-high.
2. Place the turkey into the pan—occasionally stirring—for approximately eight minutes.
3. Add the taco seasoning mix and water. Blend well.
4. Cook approximately three more minutes until the water is absorbed, and the turkey is fully cooked.

5.   Cool, and place into the corn shells with ¼ cup of the turkey each.

If desired garnish with sliced avocado or shredded lettuce.

Without the optional ingredients = 258 calories = 2 Basic tacos

Flatbread Pizza

The oven setting for this delicious treat is 450 °F.

¼ cup shredded mozzarella
¼ cup crushed tomatoes
1 whole-wheat tortilla
Basil

Instructions

1.   Put the tortilla on a baking tray.
2.   Blend the remainder of the ingredients.
3.   Bake approximately 8 to 10 minutes

The yield of 1 Serving is 270 calories.

Lunch On-the-Go: Seashell—Tomato Soup

½ Cup fresh chopped spinach
½ cup zucchini (cut into noodles, ribbons, or chopped)
1 ounce uncooked or ½ cup cooked small shell pasta (whole-grain)
½ cup marinara sauce (low-sodium such as Dell'Amore)
1 ½ tablespoons Parmesan cheese (finely grated)

1.   Prepare this as a meal on the go by using a 1-pint wide-mouth jar.

2. Layer the ingredients beginning with the sauce, noodles, and veggies.
3. Top it off with the cheese.
4. Place in the refrigerator until you are ready to eat.
5. Salt and Pepper for additional flavoring.
6. Add boiling water to the jar leaving a one-inch space at the rim.
7. Cover and steep for two minutes.

2 cups = 1 serving = 220 calories

CHAPTER 9

DINNER MENUS FOR THE INTERMITTENT FASTING PLAN

These tasty meals can be served for the entire family or savored for more than one meal.

Crab Cakes

Set the oven to 450°F.

1. Combine 3 tablespoons mayonnaise with 1 cup of crab meat.
2. Make two cakes and roll in ¼ panko.
3. Grease a baking sheet and bake for approximately ten minutes.

Total Calories: 274

Cod with Corn, Beans, & Pesto

4—six Ounce Cod Fillet pieces
1 tablespoon olive oil
2 tablespoons pesto (store-bought)
1 leek (white & light green parts)
½ Pound Green beans (2 ½ cups)
2 ears—corn kernels

Note: Leeks sliced into half-moon shapes.
Green Beans crosswise cut in halves.

Instructions

1. Preheat the oil using medium-high heat using a cast-iron skillet.
2. Flavor the fish with salt and pepper if desired.
3. Cook three to four minutes.
4. Combine the leek and beans.
5. Stir the beans and corn together and cook for one minute.
6. Blend the pesto.

Enjoy this treat for 255 total calories.

Serving Size: 4

Grilled Eggplant Salad with Halibut

2 tablespoons canola oil (add more for the grill)
4—six-ounce skinless halibut pieces
1 Medium Eggplant (Approximately 1 Pound)
1 teaspoon finely chopped fresh ginger
2 tablespoons soy sauce
1 Jalapeno (thinly sliced & seeded)
2 tablespoons rice vinegar
½ Cup fresh cilantro

Instructions

Preheat the grill to med-high.

1. Blend the oil and one tablespoon soy sauce. Cover the fish and eggplant with the oil mixture.
2. Use pre-greased grill; place the eggplant and fish on the surface until tender (approximately three to five minutes per side).
3. Combine the ginger, jalapeno, vinegar, remainder of the soy sauce, and cilantro in a small dish. Lightly sprinkle the second mixture of eggplant and fish.

Enjoy this for 301 total calories.

Serves 4

Glazed Honey Mustard Salmon

1—four-ounce salmon steak
1 tablespoon of honey
1 teaspoon canola oil
1 tablespoon Dijon mustard

Instructions

1. Preset the oven at 400°F.
2. Mix each of the ingredients
3. Use a baking dish, and add the mixture.
4. Bake for eight minutes.

Total Calorie Intake: 280

Southwestern Steak and Relish

¼ cup fresh or frozen corn
1 eight-ounce lean cut steak
1 roasted red pepper

Instructions

1. Warm up the frozen or fresh corn kernels for 1 minute in the microwave.
2. Use med-high heat to cook the steak for 8 minutes.
3. Top with the roasted red pepper.

What a yummy treat at 300 calories.

Veggie Soup

6 cups beef broth
4 cups chopped cabbage
1—28-ounce can of diced tomatoes
1 teaspoon each of oregano and basil
2 tablespoons tomato paste

Use 1-cup each of the following veggies:
Chopped zucchini
Green beans
Chopped onion
Sliced carrots

Instructions

1. Sauté the carrots, garlic, and onions for five minutes in a skillet.
2. Add the remainder of the ingredients as well as the juice with the tomatoes.
3. Simmer for one hour.
4. Flavor with salt and pepper if desired.

Note: You can use 6 cups of water and 2 onion soup pouches for the bouillon.

This one is a winner with 12 servings at 51 calories each for a 249.7 g portion.

Chicken Peperonata

125 g sliced Portobellini mushrooms
2 tablespoons olive oil
2 chicken breasts (partially boned)

2 crushed garlic cloves

1 sliced onion

250 ml Chicken stock

2 sliced Red peppers

1 teaspoon dried oregano

Instructions

1. Set the oven temperature at 375 °F.
2. Pour ½ of the oil into a skillet, flavor the chicken, and fry on each side for approximately two minutes.
3. Bake for 15 minutes in a roast pan.
4. With the remainder of the oil—fry the onion and add the mushrooms, peppers, and garlic in the skillet. Continue cooking for about five more minutes.
5. Combine the stock and oregano and add it to the mixture to and continue cooking for another five more minutes.
6. Pour the mixture over the chicken and serve.

Yields 4 Servings

Total Calorie Intake for Each Serving: 250

Light Green Bean Casserole

1 Can Cream of Mushroom (reduced fat)

2 Cups Diced Fresh Mushrooms (8 ounces)

2 Crushed Garlic cloves

6 Cups Green Beans (no salt)

½ Cup Milk 1%--Reduced fat

½ Cup French Fried Onions

Instructions

1. Set the over for 375 °F.

2. Dice the mushrooms and cut the green beans into one-inch lengths.
3. Combine the milk, soup, garlic and a dash of black pepper in a baking dish until the ingredients are well blended.
4. Blend in the mushrooms and beans.
5. Stir all of the ingredients until well mixed.
6. Sprinkle the French onions on the top.
7. Bake for approximately 30 to 35 minutes.

Yields: 8 Servings
Calorie Counts: 83.0 each

Black Bean Quesadillas

4—eight-inch tortillas (whole-wheat)
1—15 ounce can black beans
2 teaspoons canola oil
½ cup fresh salsa
1 ripe diced avocado
½ cup Monterey Jack cheese (shredded)

Instructions

1. In a medium dish—mix ¼ cup of the salsa, cheese, and beans.
2. Spread ½ cup on each tortilla—fold—press to flatten.
3. Using medium heat—pour 1 teaspoon oil and add 2 quesadillas.
4. Cook two to four minutes total (turn once).
5. Use the remainder of the oil for the other two quesadillas.
6. Serve with the rest of the salsa and avocado.

This tasty meal will feed four people with 375 calories each.

Deviled Kebabs Tofu Style

8 Small potatoes
1 tablespoon honey/clear
8 button onions/shallots
2 tablespoons soy sauce (light)
1 tablespoon sunflower oil
1 tablespoon mustard (whole-grain)
1 red pepper (without seeds and diced)
2 tablespoons tomato puree
1 courgette/zucchini—peeled and sliced
300 g (firm) smoked/cubed tofu

Instructions

1. With boiling water, add the onions/shallots in a dish to soak for five minutes.
2. Boil the potatoes for seven minutes—drain.
3. In a separate dish, combine the soy sauce, honey, tomato puree, mustard, honey, and seasonings.
4. Toss the tofu with the marinade and set for ten minutes.
5. Drain the onions from the soak and place in a pan—boil for three minutes—and drain.
6. Thread the potatoes, shallots, tofu, pepper, and courgette/zucchini on a skewer.
7. Cook them on the grill for approximately ten minutes.
8. Turn frequently and brush with the marinade before.

4 Servings
Total Calories: 178

Orange—Broccoli Tofu

6 Cups broccoli florets
1—14-ounce package water-packed tofu

1 cup orange juice

½ cup freshly chopped cilantro

3 tablespoons canola oil

1 tablespoon minced chipotle in adobo

½ teaspoon salt

Instructions

1. Drain and cut the tofu into ½ - ¾-inch cubes.
2. Sprinkle a bit of salt for flavoring on each side of the tofu (optional) if you wish.
3. Using med-high heat, use 2 tablespoons of oil and place a single layer of tofu into the pan.
4. Stir and cook for a total of seven to nine minutes—remove—and put on a dish.
5. Place the remainder of oil (1 tablespoon) to the pan and add the broccoli.
6. Cook about one minute—add the chipotle and juice—cook an addition two or three minutes.
7. Add the tofu and heat for one to two minutes.
8. Stir in the cilantro.

Additional tip: Check in the Mexican foods aisle for small cans of chipotle chilies in adobo sauce.

Serving Size: Approximately 1 ¼ cups packs 242 calories

Serves 4

www.ingramcontent.com/pod-product-compliance
Lightning Source LLC
Chambersburg PA
CBHW071241280526
45788CB00004B/1526